I0407274

A Complete Look at Adrenal Fatigue

Studies on Conditions of Subclinical Hypoadrenia

By: James M. Lowrance © 2008

ABOUT THE AUTHOR:

I am a husband, father, grandfather and lifetime contract salesman, with experience in health writing that began in 2004. I completed theological studies with Liberty University in 1996. I formerly served as editor and forum moderator of Thyroid Health for BellaOnline and as a general health writer for Suite101, where I received Editor's Choice Awards for my articles on health subjects.

In 2003 I was diagnosed with hypothyroidism; "Hashimoto's thyroiditis" being the cause. This autoimmune form of thyroid disease that causes destruction of the thyroid gland resulted in my also developing "Chronic Fatigue Syndrome", due to a compromised immune system with severe co-morbid "Adrenal Fatigue". I also suffered severe anxiety symptoms, including panic attacks early into the onset of Hashimoto's thyroiditis (Hashitoxicosis – temporary hyperthyroidism).

A Complete Look at Adrenal Fatigue

A common heart murmur I was diagnosed with in my teens called "Mitral Valve Prolapse", also worsened in severity of symptoms, with the development of these other health disorders.

My eventual receiving of diagnoses was a difficult process with proper diagnostic testing not being ordered by the first doctors I sought treatment from. These types of issues were inspiration for me to become proactive in my own health care and to self-educate myself on these health disorders, which I have done extensively since 2003. I now enjoy sharing this information with other patients experiencing my same health disorders.

TABLE OF CONTENTS:

A Complete Look at Adrenal Fatigue

CHAPTER ONE

The Common Stress Syndrome

Adrenal fatigue is a common syndrome, that in most cases is caused by chronic stress and affects a large percent of the population at some point in their lives (estimates are up to 80% of Americans), but if it can be recognized, it can also be treated.

While adrenal fatigue is not as serious as actual adrenal diseases and full-blown adrenal insufficiency, the symptoms can still be concerning and can also negatively affect a person's quality of life. With Adrenal Fatigue, as with more severe adrenal insufficient states, the hormone "Cortisol" is most commonly the one that becomes low or deficient. It is the hormone that manages stress in the body on a daily basis and provides energy for the body, in a cyclic rhythm.

A Complete Look at Adrenal Fatigue

A number of research articles going back more than 15 years, recognize mild adrenal dysfunction or a sub-clinically low functioning of the adrenal glands. This includes research articles on Chronic Fatigue Syndrome (CFS), Fibromyalgia and Post Traumatic Stress Disorder (PTSD), which have been proven in a number of medical research studies, to present with low cortisol levels. This condition, which causes characteristic symptoms (syndrome), has become increasingly common over the past several decades.

The main symptoms caused by Adrenal Fatigue, include the following.

- fatigue

- low tolerance for stress

- joint aches

- low tolerance for exercise

- irritability

- anxiety and depression

- low resistance to allergies and sicknesses

- sugar & salt cravings and over consumption of caffeine

The reason for the craving of these substances last mentioned above, is due to the need for supplying energy to the body from other sources, due to the person's adrenal glands having the diminished ability to do so.

This brings us to the understanding of what this syndrome actually is. It is a syndrome of the adrenals that have become exhausted, due to prolonged, chronic stress that has been placed upon them. The adrenal glands, which are two small glands, one sitting on each of our two kidneys, are designed to give the human body the ability to handle and spring back from stress. They do this by means of releasing hormones that circulate throughout the body, giving it coping abilities and energies to deal with stressors.

A Complete Look at Adrenal Fatigue

Stressors can be anything, mental or physical that place a demand of any kind on our bodies. This means stressors can be positive or negative but either type will place demands upon the adrenal glands.

The most important hormone released by the adrenals that help us deal with stress, is the one called "cortisol" or "cortical". It, like the hormone adrenaline, is also a "fight or flight" hormone, the difference being that while adrenaline is the hormone to help us with immediate need for increased bodily functions to deal emergencies or immediate tasks at-hand needing performed, cortical, is the long-term fight or flight hormone, that gives us a steady ability to handle all of our everyday stressors.

The hormone is also important because of its role in helping the body to convert sugar (glucose), fats, proteins and carbohydrates in-general, into energy, for ongoing use by the body.

This is actually a description of "metabolism" and other hormones in the body aid in the process as well, including the thyroid hormones. Excessively high cortisol levels in-fact can cause the manufacture of the more powerful of the thyroid hormones called the "T-3" (triiodothyronine) to be suppressed. This can, over prolonged periods of time, lead to a condition of low T3, called "Euthyroid Sick Syndrome", "Wilson's Temperature Syndrome" or "Low T3 Syndrome". This is a type of hypothyroidism that is usually temporary and will resolve on its own over time, as severe stressors are brought under control. In some cases, people with low T3 syndromes, must be given short term thyroid hormone replacement therapy, using a prescribed T3 hormone drug. This is not common but can occur in those who suffer severe adrenal fatigue or what is also referred to as "adrenal exhaustion".

CHAPTER TWO

Medical Research Confirms the Existence of Mild Adrenal Insufficiency

Stress is a known trigger for adrenal fatigue and related syndromes, such as Chronic Fatigue Syndrome and Fibromyalgia and it can also bring an autoimmune disease to the surface, that is in the body but hasn't fully manifested and thyroid diseases are some of the more common ones that are triggered by chronic stress, especially Grave's Disease/hyperthyroidism. PTSD (Post Traumatic stress Disorder) is also a chronic stress caused syndrome but is also classified as an anxiety disorder.

Adrenal fatigue and the other syndromes that have adrenal fatigue as a feature have as one proposed cause, a "blunted HPA Axis". This is referring to the group of endocrine glands that supply our bodies with needed hormones.

A Complete Look at Adrenal Fatigue

These glands are the Hypothalamus, Pituitary and Adrenals and they work in sync (axis) with each other but in these adrenal fatigue disorders, the response by these glands becomes "blunted" or slowed down, according to research that has been conducted by various medical groups.

A blunted HPA Axis is found commonly in conditions like CFS and Fibromyalgia and though some in the medical community believe this to be a bogus theory, there are many U.S. Gov/NIH medical studies to back it up. Because of this fact, adrenal fatigue syndromes should be looked at as real illnesses, with reputable medical research behind them.

Many medical doctors do not seem to be aware of these findings as mentioned above but it is referred to by several departments of the U.S. National Institutes of Health, including the CDC, NIAMS and also by studies found in The American Journal of Psychiatry.

A Complete Look at Adrenal Fatigue

What I like to point out about the medical research articles I cite in my own articles on the Adrenal Fatigue subject, is how clearly they recognize mild types of low adrenal function. The one I cite below is found on the PubMed (National Institutes of Health/National Library of Medicine) website and is among many that recognize Adrenal Fatigue type syndromes.

In the following research article link from PubMed the fact is cited that "early life stress" (ELS), can cause later-life low cortisol levels or what they term "hypocortisolemia".

Research Link>
http://www.ncbi.nlm.nih.gov/pubmed/16399913

QUOTE: *"In patients of all ages, many disorders labeled as psychiatric may actually be due to hormonal insufficiencies. ...*

For example, cortisol deficiency is rarely taken into account in a medical or psychiatric work-up, so persons with mild to moderate cortisol insufficiency are for the most part relegated to receiving a psychiatric diagnosis when, in fact, the same disorder is represented. However, the symptoms of cortisol insufficiency appear to closely parallel such psychiatric disorders as post traumatic stress disorder (PTSD) and addictions.

There has been some question of whether substance abuse causes a hypocortisolemic state. In reviewing the literature and obtaining detailed histories of addicted patients, it appears that childhood trauma, also known as "early life stress" (ELS), instead may elicit a hypocortisolemic state. This leads some to self-medicate with an addictive substance to quell the pain of a cortisol insufficiency, both physical and emotional. In fact, the literature supports the concept that addictive substances increase cortisol in predisposed patients.

Patients with a variety of psychiatric disorders including addictions were found to have signs and symptoms of mild or moderate hypocortisolemia. Generally, an appropriate comprehensive examination supported a diagnosis of cortisol insufficiency. For the most part, these patients were successfully treated with physiologic doses of bio-equivalent hydrocortisone, along with replacement of any other deficient hormone. By correcting underlying hormonal insufficiencies, many patients improved, with some patients having a total reversal of psychiatric symptoms. It is therefore reasonable to evaluate and treat hormonal insufficiencies with hormones prior to using psychotropic medication." (PubMed allows reprinting of articles for educational purposes)

This article is among many others that conclude that "stress" can be the cause of hypo-cortisolemia, cortisol being the adrenal hormone that moderates stress in the body but becomes inadequate with Adrenal Fatigue and Adrenal Insufficiency.

A Complete Look at Adrenal Fatigue

This is why I refer to Adrenal Fatigue as a "stress syndrome". Ongoing stress (chronic) can have the very same effect in taxing the adrenals as do sudden traumatic experiences (Post Traumatic Stress). Despite the obvious, there are still some in the medical community who deny the existence of Adrenal Fatigue. Are they overlooking a significant number of medical research conclusions? Apparently they are.

For many years, sources that address the Adrenal Fatigue subject (though usually referred to by other names), point out that chronic stress first elevates cortisol but prolonged demand for this cortisol output, eventually exhausts/fatigues the adrenals and cortisol levels begin to deplete. Even medical research groups are missing this point that there is first high cortisol and afterward, it becomes chronically low with chronic or traumatic stress.

Following below, is another interesting PubMed article abstract that points this fact out clearly and yet some researchers believe there is a contradiction when it actually confirms this very point in regard to cortisol first remaining chronically high and eventually falling to suppressed levels.

This research and the link, also from the PubMed website (National Institutes of Health) states that distressing events will first elevate cortisol levels but that long-term exposure to stress eventually disrupts the HPA Axis and results in cortisol levels dropping to sub-clinically low levels:

Research Link>
http://www.ncbi.nlm.nih.gov/pubmed/11068377 ?dopt=Abstract

QUOTE: *"There is a general assumption that distressing events or situations (stress) evoke the hypothalamic-pituitary-adrenal (HPA) system, with a resulting increase in cortisol secretion. ...*

A Complete Look at Adrenal Fatigue

However, our increasing understanding of the complexity of the HPA axis physiology raises questions as to the validity of this model. An increasing number of studies imply that after long-term exposure to stress, the HPA axis will eventually become dishabituated, resulting in a disruption of central regulatory systems and a net decrease of cortisol output. These findings have major implications for the interpretation of stress-induced neuroendocrine response patterns."

The preceding referenced research article gives a perfect description of what happens with Adrenal Fatigue syndromes and yet some in the medical community seem to be overlooking the obvious.

I suppose that the best thing for the time being is for the Adrenal Fatigue underground to continue informing the public until there is more widespread acknowledgment of this very real illness, that affects millions of people.

What really convinced me years ago, that mild adrenal dysfunction does exist and it has been proven in medical research, are those articles published in regard to syndromes like CFS, Fibromyalgia and PTSD (Post Traumatic Stress disorder). These articles clearly state that people with these type syndromes commonly suffer low cortisol levels and they have also found strong association of these syndromes to chronic stress, either prolonged or induced by sudden events.

Following are more example research articles and links:

This next link is to research published in 1996 by the National Institutes of health, stating that NIH researcher Dr. Straus and his colleagues found low cortisol levels in patients with CFS. They also state the fact that it has been long known that even subtle cortisol deficiency can cause lethargy and fatigue.

Research Link>
http://www3.niaid.nih.gov/news/newsreleases/1998/cfs.htm

QUOTE: "*People with CFS can suffer for years from an array of symptoms, including prolonged, debilitating fatigue, unrefreshing sleep, muscle pains, and memory and concentration problems. Although painkillers, antidepressants and other symptom-based therapies can provide some relief, specific treatments for CFS do not exist, the search for them frustrated by the unknown etiology of the illness.*

Several years ago, Dr. Straus and his colleagues found that CFS patients had slightly lower levels of circulating cortisol, the major glucose-regulating stress hormone, than did healthy individuals. Doctors havelong believed that even subtle deficiencies in cortisol can result in lethargy and fatigue. A subsequent study indicated that the low cortisol levels in the CFS patients might be due to deficiencies incorticotropin-releasing hormone (CRH), a brain chemical that helps regulate cortisol secretion.

A Complete Look at Adrenal Fatigue

To determine if they could restore the hormonal balance and thereby improve certain CFS symptoms, Dr. Straus and his former NIAID colleague, Robin McKenzie, M.D., designed a clinical trial to treat CFS patients with hydrocortisone, a synthetic form of cortisol.

... Twelve of the patients, however – all from the 33 in the hydrocortisone group –experienced significant adrenal suppression. None of an equal number of placebo recipients did.

Although the therapeutic outcome was disappointing, says Dr. Straus, we hope the results dissuade CFS patients from using a drug that potentially could cause them harm.

The fact that the treatment worked to some degree, he adds, was encouraging, but we would expect to see a greater benefit if low cortisol levels were directly responsible for symptoms of CFS."

NOTE: The article segment quotes state that cortsol supplementation (hydrocortisone therapy) showed a danger of causing "adrenal suppression", meaning there was danger for the drug to cause true adrenal insufficiency in the participants. Findings may be more favorable in future studies, should they use trials of lower cortisol doses but new studies by them, have yet to be reported.

In this next research article reference, also published by PubMed/NIH, it was concluded that both CFS and Fibromyalgia are "stress-response related" and abnormalities have been found in the "HPA Axis", the system of endocrine glands that regulate adrenal cortisol production. The study sites the fact that low cortisol has been found in patients with these stress related disorders (CFS and Fibromyalgia). They also mention in another portion of the study, not shown below, the fact that single readings of cortisol may not be sufficient in determining low cortisol levels in these patients.

A Complete Look at Adrenal Fatigue

Research Link>
http://www.pubmedcentral.nih.gov/articlerende
r.fcgi?artid=416440

QUOTE: *"We investigated abnormalities of the hypothalamic–pituitary–gonadal axis and cortisol concentrations in women with fibromyalgia and chronic fatigue syndrome (CFS) who were in the follicular phase of their menstrual cycle, and whether their scores for depressive symptoms were related to levels of these hormones. A total of 176 subjects participated – 46 healthy volunteers, 68 patients with fibromyalgia, and 62 patients with CFS. We examined concentrations of follicle-stimulating hormone, luteinizing hormone (LH), estradiol, progesterone, prolactin, and cortisol. Depressive symptoms were assessed using the Beck Depression Inventory (BDI). Cortisol levels were significantly lower in patients with fibromyalgia or CFS than in healthy controls (P < 0.05); there were no significant differences in other hormone levels between the three groups."*

Some of the other things Medical Researchers have studied in regard to CFS and Fibromyalgia, is the fact that these syndromes can have different triggers for different patients but with many, it is an underlying viral, autoimmune, bacterial etc..., type infection in the body, that causes chronic activation of the immune system and over time, this uses-up some of the adrenal reserves. The adrenals serve a major role in releasing cortisol, the body's natural anti-inflammatory, attempting to ward off inflammation.

Cortisol (also called "cortical"), is also the "stress hormone", that helps the body to deal with stresses of all kinds as previously mentioned, without it, even the smallest stressor would cause shock and death (adrenal crises). It, along with adrenaline, are "fight or flight" hormones and help protect the body from the effects of stress, from minor emotional stress, to major ones, such as a car accident or serious disease.

This next research article link is from the publishers of the New England Journal of Medicine and states the fact that low cortisol production is often associated with people suffering from Post Traumatic Stress Disorder and even by their offspring.

Research Link>
http://psychiatry.jwatch.org/cgi/content/full/2007/1210/1

QUOTE: *"Several intriguing questions are raised by the observation that adult children of individuals (especially mothers) with PTSD have the same reduction of cortisol production as do people with PTSD — even though many offspring in this group suffered from mood disorders, which typically elevate cortisol levels. If activity in the hypothalamic-pituitary-adrenal (HPA) axis is altered in pregnant women with PTSD, would their fetuses also have altered HPA function? ...*

Is a tendency toward low cortisol an inherited susceptibility marker to PTSD, and are subjects with low cortisol more likely to develop PTSD if they are exposed to a traumatic event? Do subtle changes in parenting affect the offspring's HPA activity, which is highly sensitive to environmental influence? (A previous study in rats demonstrated that early experience altered genetic expression of systems regulating the stress response.) While these questions are under exploration, a lesson for clinicians is that children of patients with PTSD (or with low cortisol) should also be evaluated for PTSD."

While, research articles do not use the term "adrenal fatigue", this is exactly what is being described by them. They will instead use terms such as "mild adrenal insufficiency", "Blunted HPA axis", "hypocortisolism" and simply "low cortisol".

These type research articles are published in significant numbers, so doctors who still do not believe that sub-clinical adrenal insufficiency exists, need to take a look at a few of these for valid confirmation of this very real syndrome.

Adrenal fatigue by whatever other name they wish to call by does exist and is found in a variety of stress-related syndromes.

CHAPTER THREE

More Detailed Symptoms of Adrenal Fatigue

If you're feeling rundown and tired and seem to have a reduced tolerance for stress, the following signs and symptoms, described in more detail, can help you recognize if it may be adrenal fatigue. A definitive diagnosis of any illness must come through a licensed medical professional.

Monitor how well you tolerate and spring back from "stressors."

While many people believe stress is always a mental side effect from too much negative anguish or mentally struggling with problems, stress is actually anything that places extra demands on the mind or body. Stress can be either positive or negative and can still result in taxing both the mind and body by lowering energy reserves supplied by the adrenal glands.

Some people refer to this as being "stressed out" and while most people experience infrequent episodes of being stressed out, if it becomes chronic from being experienced either too often or for extended periods of time, the adrenal glands may begin to diminish in their ability to help the body to cope and spring back from stressors.

The adrenal glands, two small pyramid-shaped glands that sit on top of each our two kidneys, give us these stress-coping abilities via the release of a hormone they produce called "cortisol." Many medical sources call cortisol "the stress hormone" but if the adrenal glands are overextended from relentless stress placed upon them over time, the reserves of this hormone can diminish somewhat and this leaves the mind and body less able to cope with stress. This is also why adrenal fatigue is referred to as "Low Adrenal Reserve" and "Adrenal Exhaustion."

Notice your Diet Habits - Cravings for Sugary and/or Salty Foods and Stimulants

According to many sources that address adrenal fatigue, when the adrenal glands are working at sub-normal (low) levels, the body may crave more foods containing salt and sugar because these substances will raise blood pressure and energy levels, when the adrenal glands have a diminished ability to do so. The body begins to seek ways to replace the missing energy that is usually supplied in more adequate levels by the adrenal glands. Some adrenal fatigue sufferers will also crave other stimulants, such as caffeine, alcohol and tobacco or anything that helps give them a lift in their energy levels.

The problem with this scenario of stimulant-use is that the extra stimulants will usually only act to stress the adrenals even more and will result in slowed recovery from adrenal fatigue or a worsening of it over time.

The stimulants will give the person using them a temporary energy-high but will be followed by a crash of more severe fatigue once the effects have worn off. This can create a vicious cycle of highs and lows and can also result in the adrenal fatigue sufferer having more and more dependency on stimulants, to the point that they cannot get going upon waking in the mornings without a stimulant boost (i.e. a cup of coffee) nor can they get through the entire day without repeated use of them.

If you have low stress tolerance, plus find yourself craving stimulants, including more sugary and salty foods, you may have adrenal fatigue.

Watch for Physical Signs or Changes in your Body

People suffering adrenal fatigue will find that their bodies react differently to physical exertion.

Physical exercise may become more difficult for them and they may find they do not tolerate it as well. It may also take them longer to recover from even mild to moderate physical exertion. Some adrenal fatigue sufferers will also experience mild joint and muscle aches and a vague feeling of being ill or just not feeling well.

They may also experience a condition known as "Orthostatic Hypotension," which is a slightly diminished ability by the adrenal glands to help regulate blood pressure upon standing up from a sitting or lying-down (supine) position. This condition results in blood pressure not rising as much as it normally should upon standing (in order to move the blood upward to the heart and brain). Because of this, the person will feel dizzy for a few seconds or even faint upon standing, as if they could possibly black out.

One might also feel a pressure-type sensation in their head and neck area during an episode of Orthostatic Hypotension, which is actually caused a lack of blood pressure but gives the sensation that there is extra pressure for a few seconds.

There is a medical test for detecting this condition as well, called the "tilt-table test", which consists of taking a patient's blood pressure and heart rate readings, when sitting or lying flat, then again when at various upright positions.

I – the author personally have this type of dysautonomia and it would be revealed clearly if I were to have the tilt-table test done. You can perform a home-version of this test yourself using a BP monitor, by first taking a reading while sitting, then again immediately upon standing. When I conduct this test at home, my BP drops a good 20 points and my heart rate increases 30 or more BPM.

This is too much of a fluctuation and an overreaction by the involuntary nervous system, which would also be revealed via a tilt-table test and points to an involuntary nervous system that is struggling to regulate these bodily functions (dysregulated-autonomic "dys-autonomia").

If you are found to have dysautonomia, low adrenal function can be the cause and correction of the adrenal fatigue may resolve this symptom as well as the others that have been previously listed.

Some adrenal fatigue patients have also reported that they have increased sensitivity to bright light and loud sounds and can become more irritable or jumpy in the presence of these or other physical stimuli. A combination of low stress tolerance, craving stimulants and having diminished ability to handle physical activity or stimuli, can all point to the possibility of a person having adrenal fatigue.

CHAPTER FOUR

Getting Tested for Adrenal Fatigue

Testing is important for determining whether a person has adrenal fatigue, in my opinion. I mention this because though it takes physical symptoms such as the ones previously described before a person will even want to investigate what could be wrong with them, getting the adrenal hormone levels tested is the single best indicator for adrenal fatigue and may also serve to rule the condition out.

The two hormones most commonly tested to determine a person's adrenal function are "cortisol and DHEA." These two hormones are the best indicators of how well the adrenal glands are functioning. Relatively inexpensive home, "saliva tests" are available to test these hormones and they are available online through a number of companies and are also carried by many pharmacies nationwide.

A Complete Look at Adrenal Fatigue

Saliva testing of adrenal hormones is recognized as being as reliable and accurate as blood testing by medical research groups, including the U.S. National Institutes of Health - National Library of Medicine (PubMed). If adrenal hormones are found to be low in range (normal values-reference range) or even fall slightly below the normal range, this is a more definite sign of adrenal fatigue. A result that is actually flagged clinically low should be shown to a doctor.

Keep in mind as stated earlier, that many Doctors do not recognize adrenal fatigue but will only recognize the severe type of adrenal hypo-function, called Addison's disease. Because of this, they will believe that a patient who passes a test called the ATCH Stimulation Test, which is designed to detect full blown adrenal insufficiency, needs no further investigation however, adrenal fatigue is sub-clinical (milder) and yet can still result in serious symptoms.

A patient with adrenal fatigue will pass this test, in most cases but what they actually need tested for, are the "free levels" of the major adrenal hormones - "DHEA and Cortisol".

The ACTH Stimulation Test is designed to gauge the adrenals reaction to being stimulated by the pituitary hormone ACTH, the problem is however, that with adrenal fatigue, the adrenals can be stimulated and will react but they still produce low levels of adrenal hormones consistently and they usually crash afterward from the extra stimulation because adrenal reserves are low. Being stimulated chemically from the outside as opposed having ongoing reserves, are not the same thing.

I receive e-mails often from people who suspect they might be suffering from Adrenal Fatigue and they will relate this suspicion to their Doctors. Their Doctors will usually order them a blood test of their blood cortisol level and these patients will ask me if I feel this is a good test for Adrenal Fatigue or Adrenal Insufficiency.

I usually express to them that in my opinion, blood testing needs to be the one called the "ACTH Stimulation Test", also called the "Cortrosyn Stimulation Test", which can rule out or confirm true Adrenal Insufficiency but I also point out to them that saliva testing done at multiple times during a 24 hour period, can also detect a low or abnormal cortisol rhythm as well, such as that which manifests with adrenal fatigue. I will also mention to them that a single blood draw of cortisol levels is like a snapshot reading and doesn't actually establish how well the cortisol rhythm is functioning throughout the day.

A single blood draw, of cortisol doesn't really establish what the cortisol rhythm is doing throughout the day. A better test of adrenal function in general is the "ACTH Stimulation Test" as previously mentioned, which takes a baseline reading then two more at thirty minute intervals, after giving the patient an injection of the ACTH hormone to stimulate cortisol production.

A Complete Look at Adrenal Fatigue

This is done to see if there is a significant increase in cortisol with the two stimulated readings and if there isn't an adequate response, they may diagnose adrenal insufficiency.

There are also saliva cortisol tests available that can help to establish a normal or abnormal cortisol circadian rhythm. These test kits contain tubes for collecting saliva samples at 3 or 4 different times during a 24 hour period. These are not terribly expensive and far less expensive than an ACTH Stimulation Test which may not be of concern if one has medical insurance that covers this type of diagnostic testing. Many pharmacies carry the saliva test kits, usually the "ZRT Labs, Inc." brand, so one can check with their local pharmacy for these. If they do not carry them, ZRT tests are also available for ordering online.

These are the reasons I believe saliva cortisol testing is the best method for detecting adrenal fatigue, once a patient has had full-blown adrenal insufficiency ruled out via an ACTH Stimulation test – should they first wish to take this precaution.

CHAPTER FIVE

My Personal Struggle with Adrenal Fatigue

My own ongoing battle with adrenal fatigue began to manifest several years before I experienced the onset of hypothyroidism, caused by Hashimoto's thyroiditis in early year-2003. I began to notice months previous to diagnosis of the thyroid disorder that my tolerance for stress and my recuperative abilities, to spring back from hard physical activity, illnesses, excessive stressors etc.., was slowly diminishing to a severely depleted level. When my hypothyroidism manifested, the adrenal fatigue hit a peak of severity and the combination of the two really threw me for a loop.

The first doctors I visited did not investigate to find the thyroid disease and I was not being treated for it, so in the mean time I had to push myself incredibly hard just to keep going.

I also had an extremely stressful job situation, in property management at that time and my thyroid symptoms were seriously adding to that stress.

Finally at one point, the adrenal fatigue turned into severe "adrenal exhaustion" and I experienced a strange viral-type illness that left me with a severe case of hives (these resolved over time) and swollen neck lymph-nodes that are still mildly swollen to this day. This is also the point at which my chemical sensitivities became much worse to caffeine, chocolate, alcohol and stimulants of any kind. In other words I had developed increased multiple chemical sensitivities (MCS).

I finally demanded blood tests and as a result, was treated for diagnosed hypothyroidism but the adrenal fatigue remained, re-occurring in flares of intermittent symptoms. Over time, I learned the difference between the symptoms of adrenal fatigue/exhaustion and thyroid symptoms.

A Complete Look at Adrenal Fatigue

With adrenal exhaustion, I experience severe post-exertion malaise that can take a couple of days to recuperate from, especially after hard physical activity. My low adrenal hormone levels were confirmed through saliva and urinary testing, which revealed consistently low cortisol.

I have since been treated for these health disorders and have seen significant improvement in them. I do still experience flares of adrenal fatigue symptoms, if I venture outside of a diet restricting stimulants or if I do not keep my stress levels under control.

It is my belief that CFS is strongly associated with a type of adrenal exhaustion and that adrenal fatigue can be a forerunner to it in some cases. The most well-established feature of CFS that you find in medical research (also true of fibromyalgia), are "low cortisol levels" and I do not believe this is a coincidence but something that makes sense because the main purposes of cortisol are regulating stress and controlling inflammatory responses in the body.

A Complete Look at Adrenal Fatigue

Two of the doctors I have been treated by since 2003, also diagnosed me with co-morbid CFS.

The adrenals when low functioning, cause more allergy, viral and illness responses to occur, due to the adrenals role in immune system function, being greatly diminished. Cortisol is also our body's natural anti-inflammatory and so low levels give rise to joint and muscle pain and other inflammatory reactions in the body. All of these factors combined, contribute to the symptoms of adrenal fatigue and CFS and can add to the symptom struggles of hypothyroid patients who have these co-morbid conditions.

The fact is, adrenal fatigue can be a factor in these and other chronic diseases and syndromes or not be related to anything specific otherwise.

It is important when one feels they may have adrenal fatigue, to be tested for it because other hormone imbalances and illnesses cause similar symptoms.

More pharmacies are now carrying "ZRT Labs" saliva hormone kits, including ones that test adrenal as well as the sex hormone levels.

The passion I have in the area of adrenal fatigue, besides having it myself, as part of CFS and co morbid to thyroid disease comes from the fact that far too many studies and reputable organizations recognize it, including the "Fibro & Fatigue Centers", located in 15 states, that are staffed by Board Certified MDs from just about every field of medicine, for it to still be believed to be simply a pseudo-syndrome or a psychosomatic one. This plus the fact that there are U.S. Government health studies also concluding that there are low-cortical syndromes, well establishes sub-clinical forms of adrenal hypo-function, that could all be referred-to under the term; "adrenal fatigue".

CHAPTER SIX

Treatment for Adrenal Fatigue

If you test your adrenal hormones and find that they are consistently low-normal, near borderline or even clinically low, then it would be time to check into adrenal support, first through your Doctor who will first want to test to make sure you are not experiencing full-blown adrenal insufficiency. If it is found to be the milder adrenal fatigue and not actual adrenal disease causing a more severe type of adrenal insufficiency but your Doctor does not believe in treating this lesser form, you might try finding an Osteopath or Naturopath Physician, who does recognize adrenal fatigue and the treatments that are available for it.

If these avenues for treatment by a physician are not available, you may want to purchase the over-the-counter adrenal support supplements to treat the condition yourself.

A Complete Look at Adrenal Fatigue

Should you do this, I would of course recommend taking only the manufacturer's recommended doses and that you also do some research on the support supplements you may choose to take. This would be a wise precaution, to make sure they are safe for you and that there are no contraindications that might affect you meaning; they will not interact negatively with any other treatments you may already be taking for other health issues.

Following the subheading below, are methods and treatments that can help to improve adrenal fatigue and to possibly resolve it over time.

Get more Sleep, Rest and Relaxation

In today's fast-paced society, a busy schedule can leave little time for adequate sleep, rest and relaxation. This lack of rest can heighten your stress level and place too much demand on the adrenal glands. Like any organ or gland of the body, the adrenals need time to rest and recuperate in order to rebuild their reserves and abilities to function at optimal level.

The job of these glands is to supply the body with adequate levels of adrenal hormones, but they can only do this if the body in general is allowed to rest and relax for sufficient periods of time each day.

Medical sources state that most people need a minimum of eight hours of sleep per night in order to function at their best level during the daytime and in order for the cells of the body to have adequate time to repair and restore from normal use of them. Our everyday routines also place a degree of stress upon our minds and emotions. While sleep is very important to get in adequate amounts, the same is true of simple rest and relaxation in general. If you don't allow for necessary leisure time and time to simply sit quietly or lie down and rest on occasion, you will not be allowing your body and mind to unwind from the stressors of everyday duties and this leads to that feeling of being "stressed out" by the end of the day or even before the end of the day.

Reduce your Stress Levels

No one living in the world today can escape or be immune to stress. Stress is a fact of life; our goal is to work on reducing its effects and to learn coping skills, so that we find ways to eliminate or remove as much of it as we possibly can from our lives. The adrenal glands help us to cope with and to recover from stress by providing the body with adequate levels of the stress hormone "cortisol" as mentioned in previous chapters. This hormone is also considered to be a "fight or flight" hormone, like adrenaline – the other major hormone released by the adrenals.

While adrenaline is the more short term energizing hormone needed at times of danger (to escape or fight a situation or enemy), cortisol is the long term fight or flight hormone, giving us the needed steady flow of energy, throughout the day, to perform our normal tasks. Relentless and ongoing stress can eventually use up the reserves of this hormone faster than the adrenals are able to supply it, unless we allow ourselves time to recuperate from stress.

Only then can the adrenals rebuild the reserves of this very important stress hormone and the others it continually supplies to the body.

Stress can be reduced simply by resting and giving ourselves time during each day to unwind for a few minutes at a time. It is also important not to become unnecessarily uptight throughout the day over small problems that arise. We should learn to not take the smaller problems as seriously, because there are potentially too many of them that can arise and this will keep our stress levels peaked too often and for extended periods of time.

Take Supplements that help strengthen your Adrenals

There are many supplements that can be self-administered or prescribed by a qualified physician, to help keep the body and the adrenal glands healthy and strengthened to handle the everyday stress life brings upon all of us.

A really good multi-vitamin is always a great idea and there are many good ones available, to choose from. Some major vitamin companies actually manufacture vitamins called "stress formulas" or "stress tabs" and these contain the vitamins and minerals that help the body cope-with and recover from stress.

Vitamin supplements in particular that are very helpful to the adrenal glands include the "B" vitamins – in particular, B-12, B-5 and B-6. Vitamin "C" is also an important vitamin for healthy adrenal function and also serves to help other vitamins absorb properly in the body. Minerals that can help with adrenal function include zinc, selenium and magnesium. There are also adrenal herbal formulas that contain helpful supplements such as "licorice root extract", "Asian ginseng" and "ashwagandha" but these should be researched carefully by anyone who is considering taking them as a short-term or long-term regimen and should also be discussed with your doctor before taking them. Purchasing supplements only from reliable, reputable companies is also wise.

Other natural supplements that can be taken to support the adrenals after observing the aforementioned precautions include "adrenal glandular" (usually beef source) and DHEA, an over-the-counter adrenal hormone that also acts as a precursor to sex hormones. All of these supplements can potentially be helpful, but everyone is unique and some supplements work better for some people than they do for others. Sometimes it simply takes a trial of several of these, by a process of elimination, to find the one that eventually helps the most.

Use Adrenal Steroids only under Professional Supervision

Over the past few years; I've corresponded with 100s of patients who relate the fact that they suffer severe types of "Adrenal Fatigue". They report that some of their Doctors placed them on a trial of a corticosteroid drug, which is a steroid form of cortisol, to help increase their levels of this adrenal hormone that can become constantly low in people with Adrenal Fatigue.

Cortisol is essential to our bodies in everyday functioning and in coping with everyday stressors as mentioned in several previous chapters but it also serves as an inflammatory agent in the body.

In Adrenal Fatigue patients, the trick in using safe non-steroid supplements, is to strengthen ones own adrenal glands, so that they function better in producing cortisol and other important adrenal hormones. With the more severe "Adrenal Insufficiency" (full blown), patients must be treated with a corticosteroid steroid, to replace the low cortisol as a lifelong treatment that cannot be substituted.

Treatment with corticosteroids requires strict doctor supervision and is especially true with that fact that some patient's cases are more complicated than others. Patients may be at risk for developing Cushings' Disease from prolonged use of adrenal steroids or may be on the verge of developing it, if they are not monitored closely.

In cases like these, they may also have to be tapered off of the cortisol drug, which comes in prescribed brands such as "Cortef" and "Prednisone", very slowly and if while doing so, their cortisol drops down to adrenal insufficiency level, they may need to be bumped back up on their dose again.

These facts demonstrate the importance in a medical professional being involved, who is experienced at titrating (adjusting) the steroid dose. Some patients may also have to take the cortisol steroid for the rest of their lives, even if their adrenal insufficiency began as a mild case. Certainly this does not occur in every case of adrenal fatigue that is treated with a corticosteroid and some actually see their low adrenal function improve, so that the corticosteroid eventually elevates abnormally high in their system and will need to be discontinued.

If for example, a patient develops symptoms of swelling (edema), increased appetite and weight gain while the drug is being administered, these can be symptoms of having abnormally high cortisol levels in the body, resulting in cushionoid type symptoms.

When patients are placed on corticosteroids they need follow up blood retesting and/or urine retesting of their cortisol levels, at regular intervals, similar to how thyroid hormone therapy is monitored, at two to three month intervals. If this isn't done, they can potentially develop symptoms of Cushings' Disease as previously described.

I do have a number of online articles in regard to treating Adrenal Fatigue and I don't recommend treating it with corticosteroids (cortisol steroids), whether it's the synthetic type like Prednisone or the more natural Cortef brand, unless it is a severe case that other methods and supplements have failed to improve.

The reason I discourage it for cases that are only mild to moderate, is for the very reasons I have stated. Another reason steroid treatment for Adrenal Fatigue, is not recommended, is due to the possibility of it actually progressing the Adrenal Fatigue, to full blown adrenal insufficiency. This is what occurred in patients with Chronic Fatigue Syndrome who were administered cortisol drugs in trial treatment studies conducted by the U.S. National Institutes of Health.

The studies by the U.S.-NIH and by other medical research groups have found that treating sub-clinical adrenal insufficiency syndromes, such as Chronic Fatigue Syndrome and Post Traumatic Stress Disorder, can result in further adrenal suppression. Dr. Stephen E. Straus, M.D, who is quoted in a PubMed article states; "Any time long-term steroid therapy is considered, even a low dose," he continues, "one needs to be concerned that the treatment itself may suppress the adrenal gland's normal production of steroids, which can lead to serious complications.

..." There have also been studies using smaller physiological doses that yielded promising results and that did not result in adrenal suppression in similar trials, which means it could simply be a matter of determining a safe dose level, which will hopefully be definitively determined in the near future as studies continue.

Some Doctors who do treat Adrenal Fatigue with Cortef or Prednisone, will administer it in very small physiological doses as mentioned and in so doing, can usually avoid complications, with also closely monitoring the patient's cortisol levels via repeat blood testing and by only treating them short-term until their own adrenal glands have improved. Even with this however, it carries a risk and a patient would want to be very confident in their treating Doctor.

You cannot switch from a corticosteroid also called glucocorticoids, to a simple adrenal support regimen because Adrenal Fatigue support supplements are designed to strengthen a person's own adrenal glands.

This is done so that they will begin producing their own adequate amounts of cortisol and most adrenal support, is safe enough that it can be taken lifelong, like most vitamins and minerals can.

If you are placed on a corticosteroid for Adrenal Fatigue, you'll need close supervision by your Doctor in getting better adjusted on dose or weaned off of the medication when needed. It is extremely important that you not try weaning off the medication yourself if you are being treated with the drug because this can potentially cause you to experience an "adrenal crisis", an emergency medical condition that can cause coma or death, if not treated in time.

It wasn't my intention to frighten or overly concern anyone but corticosteroid treatment is something that takes extreme caution and supervision by a Doctor and you cannot switch from such a treatment, to a different type, on your own.

If you are not confident in your current Doctor in following through with your current treatment or in tapering you off of it, I recommend seeing another highly qualified Doctor, such as an Endocrinologist for a second opinion because corticosteroid treatment is a very serious thing and you cannot take chances with it.

Incorporate Regular Exercise into your Health Regimen

Exercise is important in strengthening the body and endocrine system in general. Regular exercise also results in strengthened adrenal glands specifically. Doctors know that exercise helps hormones in our bodies to do their job better because it helps them to circulate properly and to metabolize in the system better. Cortisol, though being the stress hormone, also helps to regulate our glucose (blood sugar) and is one reason exercise helps in this process as well.

When you begin an exercise routine, it is important that you do so at the pace your body can tolerate. You do not want to overdo on exercise, whether it is the aerobic type of those for strengthening muscles. Too much exercise will not increase the benefit from it faster, but can actually have an adverse effect if not properly paced. This is especially true of people who are already experiencing adrenal fatigue. They can have reduced tolerance for exercise and if they do not pace themselves, they can worsen the adrenal fatigue rather than helping to resolve it.

Walking is one of the best exercises to start out with, and just a good everyday exercise for anyone. Some who start with walking can eventually progress to jogging, if that's what they chose at the proper time and pace. If you prefer walking as your exercise, many sources state that walking 15 to 20 minutes at least three times a week will give you a healthy benefit, and five times or more per week increases that benefit.

People with adrenal fatigue can incorporate these methods of lifestyle changes, diet and helpful, safe supplements into a daily regimen and can over time see significant improvement in adrenal fatigue symptoms. Some patients may see their adrenal fatigue completely resolve over time, using these treatment suggestions, tailored to their specific needs, which can also help to decrease the chances of the adrenal - stress syndrome from returning.

(END)

www.ingramcontent.com/pod-product-compliance
Lightning Source LLC
Chambersburg PA
CBHW060223290526
45789CB00003B/1389